28-Day Hearty Dash Diet Meal Plans & Recipes

Over 80 recipes For Weight Loss, Blood Pressure
Reduction And Diabetes Prevention

MELODY AMBERS

ISBN-13:978-1515265511

ISBN-10:151526551X

TABLE OF CONTENTS

INTRODUCTION

These days, it is dangerous to consume anything and everything that appeals to you. It is no longer just about being overweight anymore. A whole lot of health related issues like diabetes and hypertension are now on a frightening increase. It is reported that 1 in 3 Americans are hypertensive while one third are pre-hypertensive. 8.3% of people in the US have diabetes, 95% of these cases are type 2 diabetes affecting mostly children and teenagers while 79 million adults have pre-diabetes.

Enough of this gruesome statistics! The good news however is that by following the dash recipes, the risk of having high blood pressure will be lowered. An already elevated BP as well as an overweight body will also be significantly reduced.

Dash is an acronym that stands for Dietary Approaches to Stop Hypertension. It is a product of scientific research from the National Institutes of Health. It also has the support of the Heart, Lung and Blood Institute. It is an established method to gain sound health and lose weight. It is the one-stop diet plan to help in managing diabetes.

Dash recipes simply entail the consumption of lots of fruits, vegetables, low-fat dairy products, whole grains, poultry, fish and nuts. Sugary beverages, red meats and sweets are featured in limited quantities. With the dash eating plan, cholesterol and saturated fat is limited while the focus is on the increase of the consumption of nutrients such as fiber, protein and minerals like calcium, potassium and magnesium.

DASH menus that contains 2,300 milligrams of sodium helps to lower blood pressure and 1,500 milligrams of sodium in dash menus lowers it even further. This means the lower your salt consumption, the lower your blood pressure.

Although initially designed for individuals with hypertension, the DASH diet is presently recommended for anyone who wants to stay healthy.

1

How To Manage High Blood Pressure

Maintain a healthy body weight:

- Choose low -fat foods and eat smaller portions.
- Increase dietary fiber. Get 25- 35 grams of fiber every day.
- Conduct regular exercises. To maintain weight, carry out 30 minutes of daily aerobic exercise. To lose weight, carry out 60 minutes of aerobic exercise 4-5times in a week.

Eat more foods high in potassium, fiber and magnesium:

- Eat 4-5 servings a day of whole fresh fruit & 5 daily servings of vegetables. ½ cup cooked or one cup raw= 1 servings.
- Include peas, nuts, dried beans and seeds about four times in a week for magnesium, potassium and fiber.
- Choose citrus fruit 3ce in a week for fiber and potassium.

Eat more foods that contain lots of calcium:

- Choose fat-free or low-fat cheese and yogurts. Use Lactaid or lactose-reduced milk if you are lactose intolerant.

Cut down on the sodium in your meals:

- Select fresh foods.
- Do not add salt at the table. Use spices and herbs more.
- Reduce canned soups and frozen dinners with sauces.
- Avoid cured, pickled or smoked foods.
- reduce your consumption of luncheon meats such as bologna, processed turkey, corned beef, ham, pastrami and salami

Reduce caffeine:

- Choose decaffeinated tea, coffee and diet sodas.
- Do not take more than two caffeinated beverages daily even if you do have one.
- Do not take medications that contains caffeine

Drink enough fluids

- Drink at least eight cups of water every day.

Quit smoking

- If you cannot, reduce the numbers of smoked cigarettes
- Discuss with your doctor.

Take medication as directed by your doctor

- Consult your doctor if you discover any side-effects

Guidelines For Following These Dash Recipes

These dash recipes below are based on a calorie diet of 1800 to 2000 they are also based on 1 serving.

- DO NOT use salt even if included in the recipe.
- When having a pasta dish, select whole wheat pasta in place of regular pasta.
- Meals and snacks should be taken 2.5 to 3 hours apart. Do not exceed 4 hours.
- Cooked vegetables must either be steamed, grilled, baked or boiled, NEVER fried.
- Depending on the season, changes may be made to the vegetables and fruits recommendation.
- Substitute whole wheat flour for refined flour or all purpose flour when demanded by recipe.
- If you are using package products, ensure that label reads less than 10 grams of sugar and fat per serving and less than 300 mg of sodium

Be sure to consume at least:

- 4 servings of vegetables/fruits daily
- about 3 servings of whole grains daily

- about 2 to 3 servings of dairy daily

Sample Meal Schedule

Breakfast-8:00 AM

Morning snack-10:30 AM

Lunch-12:00 PM

Afternoon snack-3:30 PM

Dinner-7:00 PM

DAY ONE
Breakfast

- ½ cup of regular oatmeal with 1 tsp of cinnamon
- 1 mini whole wheat bagel
- 1 medium-sized banana
- 1 cup of low-fat milk
- 1 tbsp of peanut butter

Lunch

Chicken Breast Sandwich:
Chicken breast 2 slices (3 oz)

Whole wheat bread (2 slices)

Swiss cheese, reduced fat natural, low sodium (1 slice or 3/4 oz)

1 large leaf romaine lettuce

2 slices of tomato

1 tbsp of mayonnaise

1 cup of cantaloupe

1 cup of apple juice

Dinner

- Vegetarian Spaghetti Sauce
- 3 tbsp of Parmesan cheese
- Spinach salad
- 1 cup of spaghetti

Vegetarian Spaghetti Sauce
Ingredients:

Olive oil (2 tbsp)

Small chopped onions (2)

Chopped cloves garlic (3)

Sliced zucchini (11/4 cups)

Dried oregano (1 tbsp)

Dried basil (1 tbsp)

Tomato sauce (8-oz can)

6-oz can of no-salt-added tomato paste.

2 medium chopped tomatoes

1 cup of water

Preparation:

1. In a medium skillet, heat oil. Sauté onions, garlic and zucchini in oil for 5 minutes on medium heat.
2. Add remaining ingredients and simmer covered for 45 minutes.
3. Serve over spaghetti.

Spinach Salad Recipe:

Fresh spinach leaves (1 cup)

Grated fresh carrots (1/4 cup)

Sliced fresh mushrooms (1/4 cup)

Cooked corn, previously frozen (½ cup)

½ cup of canned pears, juice pack

Snacks

- 1/4 cup of dried apricots
- 1/3 cup of almonds
- 1 cup of fat free, no sugar fruit yogurt

Nutrients Per Day

Calories-2,078

Total fat-68 g

 Saturated fat-16 g

 Cholesterol-129 mg

Sodium-1,560 mg

Calcium-1,334 mg

Potassium-4,721 mg

Magnesium-542 mg

Fiber-34 g

Number Of Servings Per Day

Grains: 6, Vegetables: 5½, Fruits: 7, Dairy Foods: 3

DAY TWO

Breakfast

- Regular oatmeal cereal (½ cup) with cinnamon cereal (1 tsp)
- Medium-sized banana (1)
- Fat-free, no sugar fruit yogurt (½ cup)
- Low-fat milk (1 cup)

Lunch

- Tuna salad sandwich
- 1 medium apple
- Low-fat milk (1 cup)

Tuna Salad Sandwich Recipe:

Ingredients:

Tuna (drained &rinsed, ½ cup)

Low-fat mayonnaise (1 tbsp)

Romaine lettuce (1 large leaf)

Tomato (2 slices)

Whole wheat bread (2 slices)

Preparation:

1. Use a fork to break the rinsed and drained tuna apart.
2. Add lettuce, mayonnaise and tomato. Mix well.
3. Combine ingredients together and then place inside bread

Dinner

- Zucchini Lasagna
- Salad
- 1 cup of grape juice

Zucchini Lasagna Recipe

Ingredients:

Cooked lasagna noodles in unsalted water (½ pound)

Grated mozzarella cheese, part-skim (3/4 cup)

Fat free cottage cheese (1½ cups)

Parmesan cheese, grated (1/4 cup)

Zucchini (raw, sliced, 1½ cup)

Tomato sauce without salt (½ cup)

Dried basil (2 tsp)

Dried oregano 2 tsp

Chopped onion (1/4 cup)

Clove garlic (1)

Black pepper (1/8 tsp)

Preparation:

1. Preheat oven to 350°F and then spray a baking dish very lightly with vegetable oil spray.
2. Combine 1 tbsp of Parmesan cheese and 1/8 cup mozzarella in a small bowl. Set aside.
3. Combine the rest of the Parmesan cheese and mozzarella with the cottage cheese in a medium bowl.
4. Mix thoroughly and set aside.
5. Combine tomato sauce with the rest of the ingredients.
6. Spread a little layer of tomato sauce in the baking dish's bottom.

7. Add one third of the noodles in a single layer and then spread half of the cottage cheese mixture on top.

8. Add a layer of zucchini and repeat layering.

9. Add sauce (thin coating)

10. Top with sauce, noodles and the remaining cheese mixture.

11. Cover with aluminum foil.

12. Bake for 30 to 45 minutes.

13. Leave to cool for about 15 minutes.

14. Cut into 6 portions.

15. Makes 6 servings. Serving size: 1 piece

<u>Salad Recipe</u>:

Fresh spinach leaves (1 cup)

Tomatoes wedges (1 cup)

Seasoned croutons (2 tbsp)

Sunflower seeds (1 tbsp)

Whole wheat rolls (1)

Snacks

- Unsalted almonds (1/3 cup)
- Dry apricots (1/3)
- Whole wheat crackers (6)

<u>Nutrients Per Day</u>

Calories-1,988

Total fat-60 g

Saturated fat-13 g

Cholesterol-72 mg

Sodium-1,421 mg

Calcium-1,447 mg

Potassium-4,695 mg

Magnesium-553 mg

Fiber-33 g

Number Of Servings Per Day

Grains: 81/4, Vegetables: 43/4, Fruits: 5, Dairy Foods: 4

DAY THREE
Breakfast

- Shredded wheat cereal (3/4 cup)
- Medium-sized banana (1)
- Whole wheat bread (1 slice)
- Low-fat milk (1 cup)
- Fat-free, no sugar fruit yogurt (½ cup)
- Soft, unsalted margarine (1 tsp)

Lunch

- Rich Chicken Salad (3/4 cup)
- Whole wheat bread (2 slices)
- Regular mustard (1 tbsp)
- Salad

Rich Chicken Salad Recipe
Ingredients:

Skinless chicken (cooked& cubed, 31/4 cups)

Chopped celery (1/4 cups)

Lemon juice (1 tbsp)

Onion powder (½ tsp)

Low-fat mayonnaise (3tbsp)

Preparations:

1. Bake the chicken, cut it into cubes and refrigerate.
2. Add the remaining ingredients in a large bowl.
3. Combine with chilled chicken.
4. Mix thoroughly
5. Makes 5 servings. Serving size: 3/4 cup

Salad:

Tomato wedges (½ cup)

Fresh cucumber slices (½ cup)

Italian dressing (1 tsp)

Fruit cocktail, juice pack (½ cup)

Dinner

- Beef (3 oz)
- Fat-free beef gravy (2 tbsp)
- 1 cup of green beans, sautéed with:
- ½ tsp of canola oil
- 1 small baked potato:
- 1 tbsp of fat free sour cream
- 2 tbsp of cheddar cheese (natural, reduced fat, low sodium)
- 1 small whole wheat roll
- 1 tbsp of chopped scallions
- 1 tsp soft of unsalted (tub) margarine
- 1 small apple
- 1 cup low-fat milk

Snacks

- Unsalted almonds (1/3 cup)
- Raisins (1/4 cup)
- Orange juice (1 cup)

Nutrients Per Day

Calories-2,037

Total fat-59 g

Saturated fat-12 g

Cholesterol-155 mg

Sodium-1,507 mg

Calcium-1,218 mg

Potassium-4,855 mg

Magnesium-580 mg

Fiber-36 g

Number Of Servings Per Day

Grains: 5, Vegetables: 5, Fruits: 6, Dairy Foods: 2 ½

DAY FOUR
Breakfast

- Whole wheat bread (1 slice)
- Soft unsalted (tub) margarine (1 tsp)
- 1 medium peach
- Fat-free, no sugar fruit yogurt (1 cup)
- 1 cup of low-fat milk
- ½ cup of grape juice

Lunch

Ham & Cheese Sandwich:
Ingredients:

2 oz of tenderloin roast beef

1 slice of natural cheddar cheese (reduced fat, low sodium)

Whole wheat bread (2 slices)

Romaine lettuce (1 large leaf)

Tomato (2 slices)

Low-fat carrot sticks (1 cup)

Dinner

- Chicken and Spanish rice
- 1 cup of green peas, sautéed with:
- 1 tsp of canola oil
- 1 cup of cantaloupe chunks
- 1 cup of low-fat milk

Chicken & Spanish Rice Recipe

Ingredients:

Chopped onions (1 cup)

Green peppers (1/4 cup)

Vegetable oil (2 tsp)

Tomato sauce without salt (4-oz)

Chopped parsley (1 tsp)

Black pepper (½ tsp)

Minced garlic (11/4 tsp)

5 cup of rice (previously cooked in unsalted water)

3½ cups of cooked & diced chicken breast (remove skin and bones)

Preparation:

1. In a large pan, sauté green pepper and onions in oil on medium heat for 5 minutes.
2. Add the tomato sauce and spices. Leave to heat.
3. Add the cooked rice and then the chicken. Heat through.
4. Makes 5 servings. Serving size: 1½ cups.

Snack

- Unsalted almonds (1/3 cup)
- Apricots (1/4 cup)
- Apple juice (1 cup)

Nutrients Per Day

Calories-2,045

Total fat-59 g

 Saturated fat-12 g

Cholesterol-150 mg

Sodium-1,436 mg

Calcium-1,415 mg

Potassium-4,559 mg

Magnesium-541 mg

Fiber-35 g

Number Of Servings Per Day

Grains: 4, Vegetables: 43/4, Fruits: 7, Dairy Foods: 3½

DAY FIVE
Breakfast

- Currant-Apple granola
- Shake Rattle and Roll Shake

Currant-Apple Granola Recipe
Ingredients:

3/4 cup of low-fat muesli (or granola)

Fat free milk (3/4 cup)

½ of a crisp, diced medium apple

Dried currants, raisins or dried cranberries (2 tbsp)

A sprinkle of cinnamon

Preparation:

1. Combine all ingredients. Leaving the cinnamon for last.
2. Serves 1.

Shake Rattle And Roll Shake
Ingredients:

A medium banana

Honey (½ tbsp)

A shake of nutmeg

A whole peeled orange

Fat free milk (1/4 cup)

2 ice cubes

Preparation:

1. Blend all ingredients together until completely smooth
2. Serves 1.

Lunch

- Quesadillas With Smoked Shrimp
- Tasty Jicama Salad with Fennel & Tangerine
- 1 medium Pear

Quesadillas With Smoked Shrimp
Ingredients:

Grated low-fat smoked mozzarella cheese (1½ ounces)

1 diced jalapeno (optional)

3 ounces of diced cooked shrimp (or smoked chicken)

1 deseeded and chopped plum tomato

Ground cumin (½ tsp)

Diced red onion (1/4 cup)

4 or 5 cilantro leaves

Two 8-inch whole-wheat tortillas

Preparation:

1. Combine the cheese, smoked chicken or cooked shrimp, ground cumin, diced red onion, plum tomato, and diced jalapeno and mix them together.
2. Spread mixture on the tortillas.
3. In a hot nonstick frying pan, heat the tortillas for a minute or two or until it starts becoming brown.
4. Remove from pan and add the cilantro leaves.

19

5. Fold and slice into wedges.
6. Serves 1.

Tasty Jicama Salad
Ingredients:

1/4 pound of jicama

A small fennel bulb (1)

1/4 of a small red onion

 Small seedless tangerine

Salt (1/8 tsp)

A little black pepper

A tablespoon of chopped fennel leaves

Preparation:

1. Peel the jicama and then slice it into 1/4-inch thick pieces.
2. Stem, core, and halve the fennel bulb.
3. Thinly Slice ½ of it into half moon and add.
4. Thinly Slice the red onion and add.
5. Squeeze the tangerine over the fennel and jicama.
6. Sprinkle salt and mix.
7. Garnish with some black pepper and chopped fennel leaves
8. Serves 1.

Dinner

- Salmon & Ginger Sesame
- Artichoke Salad
- Whole Wheat Roll with Marmalade
- ½ cup of Sliced Strawberries
- 1 cup of fat- free Milk

Salmon & Ginger Sesame

Ingredients:

4 ounces of salmon

Soy sauce (1/4 cup)

2 tbsp of balsamic vinegar

½ tsp of sesame oil

2-inch chunk of peeled & grated ginger

Olive oil (1 tsp)

Minced green onion (1 tbsp)

Preparation:

1. Marinate the salmon in the soy sauce, sesame oil, balsamic vinegar and ginger for 15 minutes.
2. Heat a nonstick skillet briefly then coat it with the olive oil. Remove the salmon from marinade.
3. Next, sauté each side for about a minute. Sprinkle sesame seeds on the salmon in the pan.
4. Take out the salmon and garnish with minced green onion.
5. Serves 1.

Artichoke Salad

A ¼ head of chopped romaine lettuce

4 medium cucumbers (sliced)

2 ripe plum tomatoes (diced)

Artichoke hearts (4 ounces, water-packed, drained & quartered)

Small minced garlic clove

Canola or olive oil (2 tsp)

Marjoram or thyme

The juice of a fresh-squeezed medium lemon

Dried oregano (½ tsp)

Salt and pepper to taste

Preparation:

1. Toss together the lettuce with cucumber, tomatoes and artichoke hearts.
2. For the dressing, mix the garlic clove, olive or canola oil, the juice of an fresh-squeezed medium lemon, dried oregano, marjoram or thyme and salt & pepper to taste.
3. Serves 1.

Snacks

- 3/4 cup (1 oz) of Unsalted Pretzels
- 1/3 cup of Raisins

Nutritional Facts Per Day

Calories-2,039

Total fat- 45 g

Saturated fat-12 g

Cholesterol- 264 mg

Carbohydrates: 345 g

Sodium- 2, 343 mg

Calcium: 1,335 mg

Potassium-5, 201 mg

Magnesium: 344 mg

Fiber-49 g

Number Of Servings Per Day

Grains: 6, Vegetables: 6, Fruits: 6, Dairy Foods: 3

DAY SIX
Breakfast

- 1 low-fat granola bar
- 1 medium banana
- 1 cup of low fat- milk
- ½ cup of fat- free, no sugar fruit yogurt
- 1 cup of orange juice

Lunch

Turkey Breast Sandwich
Ingredients:

Turkey breast (3 oz)

Whole wheat bread (2 slices)

Romaine lettuce (1 large leaf)

Tomato (2 slices)

Low-fat mayonnaise (2 tsp)

Steamed broccoli (1 cup)

Regular mustard (1 tbsp)

Steamed broccoli previously frozen (1 cup)

Dinner

- Spicy Baked Fish & Scallion Rice
- ½ cup of previously frozen cooked spinach sautéed with:
- Canola oil (2 tsp)
- 1 tbsp of slivered almonds
- 1 cup of previously frozen cooked carrots
- 1 tsp of soft margarine
- 1 small whole wheat roll

- 1 small cookie

Spicy Baked Fish

Ingredients:

Fish fillet (1 pound)

Olive oil (1 tbsp)

Spicy salt free seasoning (1tsp)

Preparation:

1. Preheat the oven to 350°F. Get a casserole dish and spray it with cooking oil.
2. Wash the fish dry it and place in dish.
3. Mix oil and seasoning. Drizzle over fish.
4. Bake for 15 minutes. Do not cover.
5. Cut into pieces.
6. Makes 4 servings. 1 piece (3 oz) per serving

Scallion Rice

Ingredients:

4½ cups of rice (cooked in unsalted water)

1/4 cup of chopped green onions

1½ tsp of unsalted bouillon granules

Preparation:

1. Cook rice according to directions on the package.

2. Combine the cooked rice, scallions, and bouillon granules and mix well.

3. Measure 1 cup portion and serve.

Snack

- Unsalted peanuts (2 tbsp)
- 1 cup of low fat milk
- 1/4 cup of dried apricots

Nutrients Per Day

Calories-1,935

Total fat- 57 g

Cholesterol-171 mg

Sodium-1,472 mg

Calcium-1,214 mg

Potassium- 4,710mg

Magnesium- 545 mg

Fiber-36 g

Number Of Servings Per Day

Grains: 6, Vegetables: 53/4, Fruits: 5, Dairy Foods: 2½

DAY SEVEN
Breakfast

- Puffed wheat cereal (2 cups)
- 1 slice of whole wheat bread
- 1 medium-sized banana
- 1 cup of low -fat milk
- 1 cup of orange juice
- 1 tsp of soft unsalted (tub) margarine

Lunch

Beef Barbequed Sandwich:
Ingredients:

Beef, eye of round (2 oz)

Barbeque sauce (1 tbsp)

Natural, low sodium Swiss cheese, (2 slices)

1 hamburger bun

Romaine lettuce (1 large leaf)

Tomato (2 slices)

1 medium orange

New potato salad (1 cup)

Potato Salad Recipe

Ingredients:

Small new potatoes (5 cups)

Olive oil (2 tbsp)

Chopped green onions (1/4 cup)

Black pepper (1/4 tsp)

Dried dill Weed (1 tsp)

Preparation:

1. Use a vegetable brush to clean the potatoes thoroughly.

2. Boil potatoes until tender.

3. Drain the potatoes and leave to cool for 20 minutes.

4. Cut potatoes in quarters and then add olive oil, onions, and spices. Mix well

5. Makes 5 servings.1 cup, serving size

Dinner

- 3 oz cod:
- 1 tsp of lemon juice
- ½ cup of long grain brown rice
- 1 cup spinach, sautéed with:
- 1 tsp of canola oil
- 1 tbsp of slivered almonds
- 1 small corn bread muffin
- 1 tsp soft unsalted (tub) margarine

Snack

- 1 cup of fat-free, no added sugar fruit yogurt

- 1 tbsp of unsalted sunflower seeds
- Graham cracker rectangles (2 large ones)
- 1 tbsp of reduced fat peanut butter

<u>Nutrients Per Day</u>

Calories-1,955

Total fat-52 g

Saturated fat-11 g

Cholesterol-140 mg

Sodium-1,447 mg

Calcium-1,524 mg

Potassium-4,580 mg

Magnesium-598 mg

Fiber-31 g

<u>Number Of Servings Per Day</u>

Grains: 7, Vegetables: 43/4, Fruits: 4, Dairy Foods: 3

DAY EIGHT

Breakfast

- Cheese & Eggs
- ½ Whole Wheat Pita Bread Loaf
- ½ large Grapefruit

Cheese & Eggs

Ingredients:

2 egg whites

1 chopped green onion

1 whole egg

Fat free or low-fat milk (2 tbsp)

2 chopped sun dried tomatoes

Grated reduced fat extra sharp Cheddar cheese (1 ounce)

Olive oil

Preparation:

1. In a hot nonstick sauté pan already coated with olive oil Scramble egg, egg whites and milk coated with olive oil spray.
2. Sprinkle with Cheddar cheese, dried tomatoes and green onion.
3. Scramble them and place inside half of toasted pita bread.
4. Serves 1.

Lunch

- 1cup of fat free milk
- Red Peppered Couscous and Chickpeas

Red Peppered Couscous and Chickpeas

Ingredients:

1/4 cup of couscous

Warm chicken broth or vegetable stock (1/3 cup)

1 red bell pepper

Tabasco sauce   (4 drops)

Minced flat-leaf parsley (3/4 cup)

Drained, rinsed, canned chickpeas (¼ cup)

Dried apricots, diced (¼ cup)

Ground cardamom or cumin (¼ tsp)

A squeeze of lemon

Preparation:

1. Add the couscous to vegetable stock or chicken broth
2. Slice the top off the bell pepper and reserve; hollow out the pepper.
3. Dice the pepper top and then add to the cooked couscous.
4. Add the canned chickpeas, apricots, ground cardamom or cumin and Tabasco sauce.
5. Stir thoroughly and add flat-leaf parsley.
6. Squeeze the lemon into it as well.
7. Stuff the pepper and eat up!
8. Serves 1.

Dinner

- Sugar Snap sauté with Fresh Mango
- ½ cup of Low-fat Frozen Yogurt

Sugar Snap Sauté With Fresh Mango

Ingredients:

Extra firm diced tofu (1 cup) or sliced chicken breast (one 4-ounce)

Low-sodium soy or tamari sauce (1 tbsp)

Lime juice (1 tsp)

Tabasco sauce (3 drops)

A teaspoon of sugar

Sesame oil (½ tsp)

Whole sugar -snap peas, fresh whole green beans or pea pods (1 cup)

Vegetable stock or chicken broth (1/3 cup)

Cooked instant brown rice (½ cup)

Diced fresh mango (½ cup)

Minced green onions (1/4 cup)

1 tablespoon of slivered dried mango

Preparation:

1. Marinate the tofu or chicken breast in low-sodium soy or tamari sauce, lime juice, Tabasco sauce, sugar and sesame oil for about 10-60 minutes.
2. Add the tofu or sliced chicken with the marinade, the sugar snap peas, vegetable stock or chicken broth to a sauté pan.
3. Cook on high heat until the liquid is almost evaporates.
4. Add the rice, mango and onions. Stir well.
5. Garnish with the slivered dried mango.
6. Serves 1.

Snacks

- 1 medium Apple
- 6 Whole-Grain Crackers

<u>Nutritional Facts Per Day</u>

Calories-1,970

Total fat-30 g

Saturated fat-10 g

Cholesterol-325 mg

Carbohydrates: 329 g

Sodium-2,596 mg

Calcium-1, 618 mg

Potassium-3,147 mg

Magnesium-356 mg

Fiber-35 g

<u>Number Of Servings Per Day</u>

Grains: 6, Vegetables: 5.5, Fruits: 4, Dairy Foods: 3

DAY NINE

Breakfast

- 1 cup frosted shredded wheat
- 1 medium raisin bagel
- 1 medium banana
- 1 cup of low-fat milk
- 1 cup of orange juice
- 1 tbsp of peanut butter

Lunch

Salad Plate:

½ cup of tuna salad

Fat free yogurt dressing (2 tbsp)

6 fat free unsalted wheat crackers

Romaine lettuce (1 large leaf)

½ cup of low-fat cottage cheese

1 tbsp of almonds

Fresh cucumber slices (1 cup)

½ cup canned pineapple, juice pack

½ cup tomato wedges

Tuna Salad Recipe

Ingredients:

2 6-oz can tuna, packed in water

½ cup raw celery, chopped

1/3 cup green onions, chopped

6½ tbsp mayonnaise, reduced fat

Preparation:

1. Rinse the tuna, drain it for 5 minutes. Use a fork to break apart.

2. Add mayonnaise, celery and onion. Mix thoroughly.

3. Makes 5 servings, ½ cup, serving size.

Fat Free Yogurt Dressing Recipe

Fat- free plain yogurt (8 oz)

Fat- free mayonnaise (1/4 cup)

Dried chives (2 Tbsp)

Dried dill (2 Tbsp)

Lemon juice (2 Tbsp)

Preparation:

1. In a bowl, combine all ingredients together and refrigerate
2. Makes 8 servings. 2 tbsp, serving size.

Dinner

- Turkey Meatloaf
- Sour cream, low-fat (1 tbsp)
- 6 Melba unsalted toast cracks
- 1 small baked potato:
- Canola oil (1 tsp)
- 1 scallion stalk, chopped
- Cheddar cheese (natural, reduced fat, grated, low sodium, 1 tbsp)
- 1 cup of cooked collard greens (previously frozen)
- 1 medium peach

Turkey Meatloaf Recipe
Ingredients:

1 pound of lean ground turkey

Regular dry oats (½ cup)

1 large whole egg

1 tbsp of dehydrated onion

Low sodium catsup (3 oz)

Preparation:

1. Mix all the ingredients thoroughly in a bowl.

2. Bake at 350 °F in a loaf pan for 25 minutes

3. Cut into five pieces and serve.

4. Makes 5 servings.1 slice (3 oz), serving size.

Snack

- 2 tbsp of sunflower seeds

- 1 cup fat- free, no sugar fruit yogurt,

Nutrients Per Day

Calories- 2,100

Total fat-52 g

Saturated fat-11 g

Cholesterol-158 mg

Sodium-1,579 mg

Calcium-1,412 mg

Potassium-4,903 mg

Magnesium-491 mg

Fiber-31 g

Number Of Servings Per Day

Grains: 81/4, Vegetables: 43/4, Fruits: 5, Dairy Foods: 3

DAY 10
Breakfast

- Deli Yogurt With Strawberries
- Grapefruit (½ medium)
- Toasted Almonds and Granola

Deli Yogurt With Strawberries
Ingredients:

Fresh quartered strawberries (1cup)

Brown sugar (1 tsp)

Slivered toasted almonds (1/4 cup)

Low-fat granola (¼ cup)

Preparation:

1. In a cereal bowl, add the strawberries and sugar
2. Toss strawberries brown sugar and add to the middle of a cereal bowl holding yogurt
3. Top with almonds and granola
4. Serves 1

Lunch

- Rosemary Cornmeal Cake
- 1 cup of Minestrone Soup

Rosemary Cornmeal Cake

Ingredients:

1 teaspoon of olive oil

3 large cloves minced garlic

1½ cups of water

Low fat or fat free milk (1½ cups)

Salt (½ tsp)

Black pepper (½ tsp)

Crushed dried rosemary (1/4 tsp)

½ cup of instant or quick-cooking polenta

1 cup corn (frozen, canned or fresh)

Stir in 1½ ounces grated well-aged Romano cheese

1/4 cup chopped chives

Garnish with ½ teaspoon fresh minced

Rosemary (optional)

Preparations:

1. Sauté the garlic in the olive oil in a sauce pan.

2. Add water, low-fat milk, salt, black pepper and rosemary.

3. After boiling them a little, reduce heat to medium and add the polenta, stirring for about 5 minutes.

4. Once thick, add the corn and mix into the polenta. Turn off heat.

5. Stir in the Romano cheese and chopped chives.

6. Pour into a pie tin and leave it to set for about 10 minutes.

7. Garnish with some of the grated cheese or Rosemary.

8. Cut into wedges.

9. Serves 3

Dinner

- Thai Long Grilled Subs
- 1 ½ cups of Fresh Spinach and Mushroom Salad
- 1 tbsp of Vinaigrette Dressing
- 1 cup of Fresh Fruit Salad

Thai Long Grilled Subs Recipe
Ingredients:

8 minced cloves garlic

1/4 cup of fish sauce

½ zucchini

6 halved Serrano peppers

1 teaspoon of sugar

Small eggplant (½)

2 cups of vegetable stock

Juice of ½ lime

½ summer squash

2 large Portobello mushroom caps

Preparation:

1. Combine garlic, Serrano peppers, vegetable stock, fish sauce, lime juice and sugar in a bowl.

2. Slice the eggplant, zucchini and summer squash thinly.

3. Marinate these as well as the Portobello mushroom caps for 15 - 60 minutes.

4. Remove from the marinade.

5. Grill (or broil) the vegetables for 5-7 minutes on one side, checking for softness and slight char.

6. Remove the mushroom caps and then slice.

7. Layer the squash, zucchini, eggplant and sliced mushroom on toasted whole wheat hot dog buns.

Snacks

- 1 cup of low-fat Chocolate Milk
- 1 medium Banana

Nutritional Facts Per Day

Calories-2,042

Total fat-42 g

Saturated fat-.8 g

Cholesterol-34 mg

Carbohydrates: 357 g

Sodium-4,145 mg

Calcium-1,418 mg

Potassium-5,190 mg

Magnesium-379 mg

Fiber-32 g

<u>Number Of Servings Per Day</u>

Grains: 5, Vegetables: 8, Fruits: 6, Dairy Foods: 3

DAY 11
Breakfast

- Maple Oatmeal With Prunes And Plums
- Decaf Iced Latte & 1 cup of Fat- Free Milk

Maple Oatmeal With Prunes And Plums
Ingredients:

Old-fashioned rolled oats (3/4 cup)

Fat free milk (3/4 cup)

Apple cider (1/4 cup)

2 diced fresh plums

Diced prunes, peaches or dried apricots (1/4 cup)

Real maple syrup (1 tbsp)

Cinnamon or nutmeg (sprinkle)

Preparation:

1. Microwave oats in milk until it is bubbling.
2. (Alternatively, heat the milk in a sauce pan on the stove, stirring constantly and cook the oatmeal for 5-8 minutes until thickened).
3. Stir in apple cider, fresh plums, diced prunes and real maple syrup.
4. Sprinkle with cinnamon

Lunch

- Lentils with Arugula, Tomato & Feta
- 1 cup of grapes

Lentils with Arugula, Tomato & Feta

Ingredients:

Whole green lentils (3⁄4 cup)

2 large bay leaves

Water (4 cups)

Dried oregano (1 tsp)

2 large beefsteak tomatoes (scooped out)

Crumbled feta cheese (1 ounce)

Chopped arugula (1 cup)

Fresh or dried thyme (2 tsp)

Vinegar (seasoned rice or white wine, 2 tsp)

Preparations:

1. Add the lentils to water, bay leaves and oregano.
2. Simmer for 20 to 30 minutes or until tender. Drain any extra cooking liquid off.
3. Combine drained lentils, feta cheese, the diced inside of the beefsteak tomatoes, arugula, fresh or dried thyme and vinegar in a bowl.
4. Stuff the scooped out tomatoes. Garnish with nutmeg or more fresh thyme.
5. Serves 1.

Dinner

- Minted Endive & Potatoes
- Sicilian Spag and Tuna
- ½ cup of Low-fat Frozen Yogurt.

Sicilian Spag And Tuna Recipe

Ingredients:

Diced yellow onion (1/2 medium)

1 clove minced garlic

Anchovy paste (1/2 tsp)

1/2 minced chipotle Chile

Fresh chopped plum tomatoes (1 cup)

Capers (drained and rinsed (1 tsp)

Chopped fresh spinach (1 cup)

Fresh tuna or canned, packed in water (3 ounces)

Fresh or dried marjoram (1/2 tsp)

Whole wheat spaghetti (2 ounces)

Preparations:

1. In a hot nonstick pan, sauté the onion, garlic, anchovy paste, and chipotle chile for 2 minutes.
2. Add the plum tomatoes, capers and sauté for 2 minutes.
3. Add the spinach and tuna cut in cubes of 1/2 inch cubes. Cook for 1-2 minutes. Turn off the heat.
4. Sprinkle with marjoram. Serve over wheat spaghetti. Serves 1.

Minted Endive & Potatoes Recipe

Ingredients:

2 large cloves of slivered garlic

Olive oil (1tsp)

Endive, leaves and bottoms (2 cups)

Red skin new potatoes (1/4 pound)

Ground black pepper (1/4tsp)

Slivered mint (1/4 cup)

Chicken stock (1/2 cup)

Preparation:

1. To a hot saucepan, add the slivered garlic and sauté in olive oil for 10 seconds.
2. Add the potatoes and endive leaves and bottoms. (2 inches trim bottom cut into 1-inch pieces).
3. Sauté for about 2minutes until endive is wilted.
4. Add pepper, slivered mint and chicken stock.
5. Cover for 5 minutes and simmer.
6. Serves 1.

Snack

- 1/4 cup of dried fruit mixture (1 oz)
- 6 Whole-Grain Crackers

Nutritional Facts Per Day

Calories-2,043

Total fat-26 g

Saturated fat-8 g

Cholesterol-86 mg

Carbohydrates: 359 g

Sodium-2, 725 mg

Calcium-.1, 255 mg

Potassium- 5, 229 mg

Magnesium-325 mg

Fiber- 58 g

Number Of Servings Per Day

Grains: 4.5, Vegetables: 9, Fruits: 4, Dairy Foods: 3

DAY 12
Breakfast

- Peppered Hash Brown Potatoes With Scrambled Eggs
- 1 medium Orange
- Whole-Grain Toast
- Decaf Caffe Latte and 1 cup of fat- free Milk

Peppered Hash Brown Potatoes With Scrambled Eggs
Ingredients:

2 small red-skinned new potatoes

Yellow onion (1⁄4 medium)

Green bell pepper (1⁄4)

Olive oil (1 tsp)

Salt (1⁄4 tsp)

Pepper (1⁄4 tsp)

Rich vegetable stock or chicken broth (1⁄4 cup)

1 whole egg

1 egg white

Fat- free milk (1 tsp)

Preparation:

1. Pre-heat a large skillet over medium high heat. Cut potatoes, pepper and yellow onion into 1⁄2 -inch pieces.
2. Sauté them in olive oil. Season with salt and pepper. Stir for 8-10 minutes or until brown.
3. Add rich vegetable stock or chicken broth. Cover for 3 minutes.

4. Separately, whisk whole egg, egg white and fat free milk together.
5. Reduce heat to low, and then pour the eggs into the vegetables while stirring.
6. Cook for about 20 minutes or until firm.
7. Serves 1.

Lunch

- Spicy Black Bean Corn Soup
- 6 Baked Tortilla Chips
- Cool Spicy Orange and Cucumber Salad
- 1 cup of fat- free milk

Spicy Black Bean Corn Soup
Ingredients:

1/4 small diced white onion

1/2 small deseeded and diced poblano pepper

2 cloves minced garlic

Cumin (1/4 tsp)

Dried oregano (1/4 tsp)

Olive oil (1/2 tsp)

Drained, rinsed black beans (15-ounce can)

1/2 cup frozen or fresh corn

Balsamic vinegar (1 tsp)

Well-aged grated parmesan cheese (1 tsp)

Preparation:

1. Sauté white onion, poblano pepper, minced garlic, dried oregano and cumin powder in olive oil for 2 minutes over high heat.
2. Add black beans, corn, balsamic vinegar and chicken stock.
3. Simmer for 5-8 minutes. Top with parmesan cheese.
4. Serves 1.

Cool Spicy Orange and Cucumber Salad
Ingredients:

A squirt of lime

A whole orange

1/2 large cucumber

Chili powder (1/4 tsp)

Toasted pumpkin seeds (1 tsp)

Preparation:

1. Slice cucumber and orange.
2. Sprinkle with lime, chili powder and pumpkin seeds.
3. Serves 1.

Dinner

• Mexican Chicken with olives & Raisins

• Melon Balls, 1 cup

Mexican Chicken With Olives & Raisins Recipe

Ingredients:

Uncooked long grain rice (1/4 cup)

Olive oil (1 tsp)

Any flavorful salsa (½ cup)

Chicken stock (½ cup)

Halved chicken breast

Baby carrots (3/4 cup)

Pitted Chopped Green Olives (2 tbsp)

Ground cinnamon (1/2 tsp)

Dark raisins (2 tbsp)

Chopped parsley or cilantro (2tbsp)

Preparation:

1. In a 6-quart pan, sauté the rice in olive oil for 2 minutes or until the rice pops.
2. Add the salsa, baby carrots, green olives, dark raisins and ground cinnamon.
3. Bring to simmer, stirring once.
4. Cover and bake in a 375 degree oven for about 25 minutes until the stock is absorbed.
5. Sprinkle parsley or cilantro and mix together with a fork.
6. Serves 1.

Snack

• 1 cup of fat-free Yogurt,

• 1 ½ cup of microwave popcorn, plain

DAY 13
Breakfast

Sunrise Blueberry Pancakes

1 cup of fat free milk

1 tsp of honey

Sunrise Blueberry Pancakes Recipe
Ingredients:

All-purpose flour (1 cup)

Low-fat or nonfat buttermilk (1 1/3 cups)

Baking powder (2 tsp)

Baking soda (1/4 tsp)

Salt (1/4 tsp)

Sugar (1 tsp)

Egg substitute (1/4 cup)

Vegetable oil (1 tsp)

Frozen blueberries (½ cup)

Cooking spray

Preparation:

1. In a large bowl, combine the flour, baking soda, baking powder, salt and sugar.
2. In another bowl, combine the egg substitute, buttermilk and oil and add to the dry ingredients.

3. Stir until the dry ingredients are moistened. Add the blueberries and stir.
4. Pour 1/4 cup batter onto skillet previously coated with cooking spray for each pancake.
5. The pancake is ready when edges looked cooked and tops are bubbly.
6. 12 servings (serving size:1 pancake)

Lunch

Pineapple And Chops With Chili Slaw
Ingredients:

Boneless top loin pork chops (8 ½ -inch cuts)

Chili powder (1-½ tsp)

Sliced cored fresh pineapple (½)

Cider vinegar   (3 Tbsp)

Orange juice (2 Tbsp)

Olive oil (2 Tbsp)

Sugar (1 Tbsp)

Cored and sliced small green cabbage (5 cups)

Thinly sliced red onion (½)

Red sweet pepper (1 small one, cut in strips)

Preparation:

1. Sprinkle salt and 1 tsp of chili powder on the chops.
2. Preheat gas grill, reduce heat to medium and then grill pineapple and chops, covered.
3. For chili slaw, whisk the sugar, juice, oil, vinegar and the rest of the half tsp of chili powder together.
4. Add sweet pepper, onion and cabbage and toss.

5. Season with salt and pepper.
6. Serve the chops with slaw and pineapple pieces.
7. Serves 4

Dinner

Chicken &Tofu Stir Fry
Ingredients:

Olive oil (2 tbsp)

Orange juice (2 tbsp)

Reduced-sodium soy sauce (1 tbsp)

Worcestershire sauce (1 tbsp)

Grated fresh ginger (1 tbsp)

Dry mustard (1 tbsp)

Ground turmeric (1 tbsp)

Cooked chicken breast, cubed (8 oz)

Extra-firm drained and cubed tofu (fresh bean curd, 8 oz)

Celery, bias slice (2 stalks)

Pea pods (1 cup) and/or sliced fresh mushrooms

3 green onions cut into ½ -inch-long pieces

1 medium red and/or green sweet pepper, cut into thin bite-size strips

Chopped baby bok choy and/or fresh bean sprouts (2 cups)

Hot cooked brown or white rice (3 cups)

Preparation:

1. Add 1 tablespoon of the oil, soy sauce, the orange juice, ginger, turmeric, Worcestershire sauce and mustard in a large bowl and stir together.
2. Add the chicken, the tofu and then stir to coat. Cover bowl and allow chilling for about 4 hours.
3. Heat the remaining 1 tsp oil over medium-high heat in a large non-stick skillet.
4. Add the celery, stir and cook for 2 minutes.
5. Add mushrooms and/or pea pods; stir and cook for 2 minutes.
6. Add sweet pepper and green onion; cook and stir for 2 minutes
7. Stir in bean sprouts and/or bok choy. Add the un-drained chicken mixture. Let it heat.
8. Serve recipe with hot cooked rice.
9. Makes 6 (1 cup stir-fry plus ½ cup rice)

Snacks

Roasted Pepper Rolls
Ingredients:

Reduced-fat cream cheese, softened (½ of an 8-ounce package)

Soft goat cheese (4 ounces)

Fat-free milk (1 tbsp)

1 small minced clove garlic

Freshly ground black pepper (1/4 tsp)

Roasted red sweet peppers, drained chopped (½ cup)

Snipped fresh basil (1/4 cup)

8 8-inch whole wheat or plain flour tortillas

Packed fresh spinach leaves (2 cups)

Preparation:

55

1. For filling, in a medium bowl, use an electric mixer to beat cream cheese for 30 seconds on medium to high speed. Add black pepper, goat cheese, milk and garlic. Beat until smooth. Add red peppers and basil, stir.
2. To assemble, divide the filling among tortillas and spread to within ½ inch of the edges. Arrange the spinach leaves over filling so its covers. Carefully roll up tortillas tightly. Cover the rollup and chill it for 3 to 24 hours. Place with ice packs in an insulated container.
3. To serve, cut roll-ups crosswise into 48 pieces with a knife. Makes 24 servings

DAY 14
Breakfast

- 3/4 cup of whole grain cereal
- 1 cup of fat-free milk

Lunch

Raspberry- Cranberry Spinach Salad
Ingredients:

Frozen red raspberries in syrup, thawed (1 10-ounce package)

Sugar (1/4 cup)

Cornstarch (2 tsp)

Cranberry-raspberry juice cocktail (½ cup)

Red wine vinegar (1/4 cup)

Celery seed (1/4 tsp)

Ground cinnamon (1/4 tsp)

Ground cloves (1/8 tsp)

Fresh spinach stems (1 10-ounce package)

Broken walnuts (1/3 cup)

Dried cranberries (1/4 cup)

Sunflower seeds (2 tsp)

3 thinly sliced green onions

Preparation:

1. For dressing, in a food processor or a blender cover and process or blend raspberries until smooth. Remove seeds by using a sieve to strain. Discard seeds.
2. Stir together cornstarch and sugar in a medium saucepan. Add the strained raspberries and stir over medium heat until it is bubbly and thickened. Cook for another 2 minutes.
3. Transfer it to a nonmetal container. Cover and leave to chill until serving time.
4. To serve, toss together, walnuts, spinach, sunflower seeds, dried cranberries and green onions in a salad bowl. Drizzle of the dressing over it.
5. Cover and chill the remaining dressing for about a week for use in other fruits or vegetable salads.

Dinner

Cornish Game Hen & Roasted Root Vegetables
Ingredients:

1 medium carrot (cut into large chunks)

1 medium russet potato (cut into large chunks)

1 medium parsnip or turnip (peeled & cut into large chunks)

1 small onion, quartered

Olive oil (1 tbsp)

Balsamic vinegar (1 tbsp)

1 Cornish game hen or poussin (about 1½ pounds)

2 minced cloves garlic

Snipped fresh rosemary (2 tbsp) or crushed dried rosemary (½ tsp)

Salt (1/4 tsp)

Coarsely ground black pepper (1/8tsp)

Pear-shaped cherry tomatoes (optional)

Fresh rosemary or sage leaves (optional)

Preparation:

1. Begin by preheating oven to 400 degree F. combine carrot, parsnip or turnip, onion and potato in a large bowl. Add balsamic vinegar and oil; toss to coat lightly. Spread in a baking pan and cover with foil.
2. Roast for 25- 30 minutes. Reduce the oven temperature to 375 degree F.
3. Meanwhile, separate the skin from the hen breast as well as tops of drumsticks very gently by using your fingers or a paring knife between the skin and the meat. Make 2 pockets extending down to the neck cavity as well as over the drumsticks.
4. Combine rosemary, garlic, salt & pepper in a small bowl. Set aside 1 tsp of the fresh rosemary mixture (½ teaspoon for dried rosemary). Rub the rest of the rosemary mixture under the skin onto the drumsticks and breast. Use a cotton string to tie the drumsticks to tail and the wing tips to body.
5. Sprinkle the remaining rosemary mixture on the skin. Leave the vegetables open. Add hen to the baking pan.
6. Uncover hen and vegetables and roast until vegetables are tender and a thermometer inserted into the hen's thigh (without touching the bone) registers 180 degree F.
7. Stir vegetables. Remove the string. Cover with foil and allow it to stand for 10- 12 minutes before serving.
8. Garnish with sage leaves and tomatoes or fresh rosemary if desired. Use a long heavy knife or shears to cut the hen lengthwise in half, remove skin and serve with vegetables. Serves 2.

Snacks

Berries Yogurt Pops

½ sandwich (Whole wheat bread, lettuce, tomato,

& low- sodium turkey lunch meat)

Berries Yogurt Pops Recipe

Ingredients:

Low-fat vanilla yogurt (2 cups)

Assorted berries (such as chopped strawberries, blackberries, raspberries, blueberries, 1 cup)

5 halved pretzel rods or 10 baked snack stick crackers

Preparation:

1. Gently stir the yogurt and fruit together in a large bowl. Spoon into 3-ounce paper cups or 4-ounce ice-pop molds. Cover the molds or cups with foil.
2. Using a sharp knife, cut a little hole in the foil and insert cut side of snack stick or pretzel rod. Freeze until it is firm. Remove foil and mold before serving.
3. Store for 1 month. Makes 6 pop

DAY 15
Breakfast

- ½ cup of 100% juice (no sugar added)
- Southwestern Morning Bake

Southwestern Morning Bake
Ingredients:

Black beans, rinsed and drained (1, 15-ounce can)

Canned enchilada sauce (3/4 cup)

2 diced, drained green chile peppers, drained

Thinly sliced green onions (½ cup)

Dashes of bottled hot pepper sauce (optional)

2 minced cloves garlic, minced

1 cup of shredded Monterey Jack cheese and/or shredded sharp cheddar cheese with jalapeno peppers (4 ounces)

3 egg yolks

3 egg whites

All-purpose flour (2 tbsp)

Salt (1/4 tsp)

Milk (½ cup)

Snipped fresh cilantro (1 tbsp)

Bottled salsa (optional)

Dairy sour cream (optional)

Preparation:

1. Grease baking dish and then combine green chile peppers, black beans, enchilada sauce, garlic green onions and hot pepper sauce (optional). Sprinkle with cheese.
2. Using an electric mixer, beat egg whites in a mixing bowl on medium speed until the tips curl. Set aside.
3. Combine flour, egg yolks and salt in a large bowl. Use a wire whisk to beat mixture until well combined.
4. Gently whisk in milk until it becomes smooth. Fold the cilantro and beaten egg whites into egg yolk mixture.
5. Pour the egg mixture carefully over the bean mixture in baking dish.
6. Bake at 325 degrees until egg mixture looks set when shaken gently. Allow for 15 minutes before serving.
7. Serve with salsa, sour cream, and extra snipped fresh cilantro if desired. Makes 8 servings

Lunch

Italian Green Beans and cheese with Penne Salad
Ingredients:

Dried penne or other short pasta (6 ounces)

1 tbsp of snipped fresh tarragon or ½ teaspoon of crushed dried tarragon

Fresh Italian green beans, cut into 1-inch pieces (8 ounces) or frozen Italian green beans, thawed (9-ounce)

1/3 cup of fat-free Italian salad dressing

Fresh shredded spinach leaves (4 cups)

Torn radicchio (2 cups) or finely shredded red cabbage (1 cup)

Freshly ground black pepper (½ tsp)

Crumbled Gorgonzola cheese (½ cup, 2 ounces)

Preparation:

1. Cook pasta following package direction. At the last 5 to 8 minutes of cooking, add fresh green beans to pasta. (If using frozen and thawed beans, add at the last 3 to 4 minutes.)
2. Rinse the pasta and beans thoroughly under cold running water and then drain completely.
3. Combine Italian dressing, pepper and tarragon in a large mixing bowl. Add beans, pasta and cabbage or radicchio. Gently toss to coat.
4. Serve on a bed of shredded spinach. Top it with the Gorgonzola cheese.
5. Makes 8 side-dish servings.

Dinner

Pork Slice With Pear-Maple Sauce

Pork tenderloin (1, 12 to 16-ounce)

Snipped fresh rosemary (2 tsp) or crushed dried rosemary (½ tsp)

Snipped fresh thyme (1 tsp) or crushed dried thyme (1/4 tsp)

Salt (1/4 tsp)

Black pepper (1/4 tsp)

Olive oil or cooking oil (1 tbsp)

Dried tart red cherries, halved (2 tbsp)

2 medium peeled & coarsely chopped pears

Maple-flavored syrup pure maple syrup (1/4 cup)

Apple juice or dry white wine (2 tbsp)

Preparation:

1. Remove fat from meat and cut into 1/4-inch slices. Combine thyme, rosemary, pepper and salt in a medium bowl. Add meat slices and toss to coat.
2. In a large pan cook meat in hot oil, half at a time until slightly pink in center. Turn only once. Remove from pan and set aside.
3. In the same pan combine pears, dried cherries, white wine and maple syrup. Bring to boiling and reduce heat. Boil uncovered for about 3 minutes. Return meat to pan with pears. Heat through.
4. Using a slotted spoon, transfer the meat to a warm serving platter. Pour the mixture over the meat.
5. Makes 4 servings.

Snack

1 oz of almond

½ Grapefruit

DAY 16
Breakfast

- Golden Brown Granola
- 1 cup of fat-free milk
- 1 cup of watermelon

Golden Brown Granola Recipe
Ingredients:

Regular oats (3 cups)

Sliced unblanched almonds (3/4 cups)

Honey (½ cups)

Canola or vegetable oil (1 tbsp)

Cinnamon (1 tsp)

Salt (1/8 tsp)

Ground cloves (1/8 tsp)

Wheat bran flakes cereal (3 cups)

Dried mixed fruit or golden raisins (3/4 cups)

Preparation:

1. Begin by preheating oven to 325°. Then spread almonds and oats on an ungreased baking sheet in a single layer.
2. Bake for 10 minutes. Stir properly. Continue baking until it is lightly toasted, that is about 5 minutes.
3. Meanwhile, in a large bowl, combine the cinnamon, honey, salt, oil and cloves.
4. Add the warm and toasted oat mixture to bowl and then toss well. Use parchment paper or cooking spray to line or coat the previously used baking sheet.

5. Place the mixture back to the pan. Bake until golden brown. Leave it on the pan to cool completely on a wire rack.
6. Break oat mixture into chunks. Toss with cereal and raisins. Cover tightly
7. Store at room temperature for 2 weeks.

Lunch

Brussels Sprouts &Toasted Almonds
Ingredients:

Fresh Brussels sprouts (2 pounds)

Olive oil (2 tbsp)

Reduced-sodium chicken broth (1 14-ounce can)

Butter (2 tbsp)

Ground black pepper (3/4 tsp)

Salt (1/4 tsp)

Sliced toasted almonds (1/3 cup)

Preparation:

1. Trim stems and take out any wilted outer leaves from the Brussels sprouts. Wash the sprouts.
2. Halve the Brussels sprouts and then heat oil over medium heat in a large skillet.
3. Add Brussels sprouts and cook until golden brown. Stir occasionally.
4. Add broth to sprouts. Bring it to boiling; reduce the heat then cover. Allow to simmer for 5 minutes.
5. Uncover it and leave to simmer until sprouts are tender and most of the liquid has evaporated. Stir occasionally. Add salt, butter and pepper, stirring until sprouts are fully coated.

6. Gently stir in the toasted sliced almonds. Serve warm.
7. Makes 12 (about ½ -cup) servings.

Dinner

½ Cup of Cooked Brown Rice

Lime-Peppered Fish With Cucumbers
Ingredients:

Frozen or fresh skinless, boneless fish e.g. sea bass cusk or swordfish (1 pound)

Dry white wine (1/4 cup)

Chicken broth (1/4 cup)

Lime juice (2 tbsp)

Cornstarch (2 tsp)

Honey (1 tsp)

Ground ginger (1/4 tsp)

Ground coriander (1/4 tsp)

Cooking oil (1 tsp)

Pepper (1/8 tsp)

Nonstick spray coating

2 medium-sized seeded cucumbers or zucchini (cut into 2x½ inch sticks)

Red or green sweet pepper (1 cut into 3/4-inch squares)

Preparation:

1. Cut fish into 3/4-inch pieces and then set aside. Thaw if frozen.

2. For sauce, stir chicken broth, wine, cornstarch, ginger, honey, lime juice, coriander and pepper   together. Set aside.
3. Spray nonstick spray coating on a large skillet then preheat the skillet on medium-high heat.
4. Add the cucumbers and stir-fry 1 to ½ minutes.
5. Add red or green pepper. Stir-fry again until crisp-tender. Remove from skillet.
6. Add half of the fish to skillet and stir-fry until fish flakes easily when it is tested with a fork. Remove.
7. Add oil to hot skillet. Add the rest of the fish and stir-fry until fish flakes easily when it is tested with a fork. Place all fish back to skillet. Push fish from middle of skillet.
8. Stir the sauce and add it to center of skillet. Cook and stir until it is thickened and bubbly. Return the vegetables to wok. Stir ingredients together so it coats with sauce
9. Cook for 1 minute, stirring well. If desired, serve with lime wedges.
10. Makes 4 servings.

Snack

½ avocado

1 medium banana

DAY 17
Breakfast

- Warmed fruity Peaches
- 1 cup of fat-free milk

Warmed fruity Peaches Recipe
Ingredients:

4 halved and pitted peaches

Dried tropical mixed fruit (½ cup)

Toasted slivered almonds (1/4 cup)

Graham cracker crumbs (2 tbsp)

Brown sugar (2 tbsp)

Ground allspice (1/4 tsp)

Peach nectar (1 can, 12-ounce)

Vanilla yogurt, divided (½ cup)

Preparation:

1. Preheat oven to 350°.
2. Scoop peach pulp out so it forms a 2-inch circle in the middle of each half.
3. Reserve the pulp and thinly chop.
4. Combine pulp, toasted almonds, dried fruit, allspice, graham cracker crumbs and brown sugar.
5. Divide the pulp mixture among peach halves evenly.
6. Place peach halves in a baking dish. Add nectar to pan and bake at 350° until the peaches are tender.
7. Use the liquid from pan to drizzle the peach halves evenly.
8. Top well with yogurt.
9. 8 servings (serving size: 1 peach half plus 1 tbsp yogurt) servings

Lunch

Cabbage- Chicken Mix

Ingredients:

4 medium-sized skinless boneless chicken breast halves (1 pound in all)

Cooking oil (1 tablespoon)

Shredded green cabbage (4 cups)

Shredded red cabbage (4 cups)

Shredded Napa cabbage (4 cups)

Finely shredded lemon peel (1 tablespoon)

Salt (1 teaspoon)

Pepper (3/4 teaspoon)

Preparation:

1. Cut the chicken into thin strips. Next, heat oil over medium-high heat in large skillet.
2. Add half of the chicken to the hot skillet. Stir-fry until no pink remains or for 2 to 3 minutes. Remove the chicken. Repeat with the rest of the chicken. Cool chicken slightly.
3. In a large bowl, combine chicken, lemon peel cabbages, salt, and pepper. Toss gently to mix well.
4. Makes 6 servings.

Dinner

Tropical Smoked Chops

Mixed Green Salad

Tropical Smoked Chops

Ingredients:

Pork loin chops (4, cut 1½ inch thick)

Jamaican jerk seasoning (2-3 tsp)

Pecan or cherry wood chunks (6- 8)

1 medium mango (peeled, seeded, and chopped, about 1 cup)

1/4 cup of sliced green onion

Snipped parsley or fresh cilantro (2 tbsp)

Jamaican jerk seasoning (1/4 tsp)

Finely shredded orange peel (½ tsp)

Orange juice (2 tsp)

Fresh cilantro or parsley sprigs (optional)

Preparation:

1. Soak the wood chunks in water at least an hour before smoke cooking. Drain water before using.
2. Trim the fat from chops. Next, evenly sprinkle the 2- 3 teaspoons jerk seasoning over chops and then use your fingers to rub it in.
3. Arrange drained wood chunks, preheated coals and water pan in a smoker. (Follow the manufacturer's directions).
4. Pour water into the pan. Place the chops on the grill rack over water pan and then cover.
5. Smoke at 160 degrees until the juices run clear.
6. Meanwhile, in a medium bowl, stir mango, orange juice, green onion, the 1/4 teaspoon jerk seasoning, cilantro and orange peel. Allow to stand for 15 to 20 minutes at room temperature in order to blend flavors.
7. Serve this sauce over chops. Garnish chops with cilantro sprigs if desired.

8. Makes 4 servings

Snack

Quick Oatmeal Cookies
Ingredients:

½ cup of softened butter or margarine

1/3 cup of packed brown sugar

1/3 cup of granulated sugar

½ tsp of vanilla

½ cup of reduced-fat peanut butter

1 cup of quick-cooking rolled oats

½ tsp of baking soda

1 cup of all-purpose flour

2 egg whites

Preparation:

1. Add peanut butter and butter in a large mixing bowl. Use an electric mixer to beat them on medium to high speed until thoroughly combined.
2. Add baking soda, granulated sugar and brown sugar. Beat until well combined, occasionally scraping sides of bowl.
3. Beat in vanilla and egg whites until mixed. Beat in as much flour as possible with the mixer. Stir any remaining flour in. Stir in oats.
4. Use rounded teaspoons to drop dough on ungreased cookie sheets by 2 inches apart. Bake for 7 to 8 minutes in a 375 degree F oven or until the edges are golden. Leave it for 1 minute to cool on cookie sheet.
5. Transfer to a wire rack for final cooling. Makes 40 cookies.

DAY 18
Breakfast

- 3/4 cup of whole grain granola cereal
- ½ cup of cantaloupe
- 1 cup of fat-free milk

Lunch

Tortellini-Veg Salad
Ingredients:

Refrigerated cheese tortellini (1, 9-ounce)

Sliced fresh mushrooms (1 ½ cups)

Torn mixed greens (6 cups)

1 medium-sized red or yellow sweet pepper (cut into strips, 1 cup)

Snipped fresh basil (1/4 cup)

White wine vinegar or white vinegar (1/4 cup)

Water (2 tbsp)

Olive oil (2 tbsp)

Sugar (2 tsp)

2 minced cloves garlic

Ground black pepper (1/4 tsp)

Toasted garlic-and-onion croutons, fat-free (½ cup)

Preparation:

1. Following the package instructions, cook the tortellini in a saucepan but do not add oil and salt. Drain it and then rinse it with cold water. Drain again.
2. Combine tortellini, basil, sweet pepper, mixed green and mushrooms in a large bowl.
3. In a screw-top jar, combine the black pepper, white wine vinegar, sugar, garlic and oil. Cover and shake well. Pour this combination over the tortellini mixture. Coat by tossing.
4. Divide tortellini mixture among four serving plates.
5. Top with croutons.
6. Makes 4 main-dish servings.

Dinner

Quinoa With Smoked Tofu Salad
Ingredients:

Water (2 cups)

Salt, divided (3/4 tsp)

Quinoa (1 cup)

Extra-virgin olive oil (3 tbsp)

Freshly ground pepper (1/4 tsp)

Lemon juice (1/4 cup)

2 small minced cloves garlic

Package baked smoked tofu, diced (1 6- or 8-ounce)

Chopped fresh parsley (½ cup)

1 cup of halved grape tomatoes

1 small diced yellow bell pepper

1 cup of diced cucumber

Chopped fresh mint (½ cup)

Preparation:

1. In a medium saucepan, bring water and ½ tsp of salt to boil. Add the quinoa and bring it back to boil.
2. Reduce to a simmer, cover it and cook for15 to 20 minutes or until water is absorbed.
3. On a baking sheet, spread the quinoa and leave for 10 minutes to cool.
4. Meanwhile, get a large bowl and whisk garlic, lemon juice, the remaining 1/4 tsp of salt, oil and pepper in it.
5.   Add the cooled quinoa, bell pepper, tomatoes, tofu, cucumber, mint and parsley. Toss properly to combine.
6. makes 6 (about 1 1/3 cups each)servings

Snacks

½ cup of non- fat fruit yogurt

½ cup of grapes

DAY 19
Breakfast

- 3/4 cup of whole grain cereal
- 1 cup of fat-free milk
- 1 cup of berries

Lunch

Lemony Pork Salad
Ingredients:

Pork tenderloin (1 pound)

Finely shredded lemon peel (1 tbsp)

6 leaves of thinly sliced fresh sage

Ground cumin (½ tsp)

Ground black pepper (1/4 tsp)

Chopped tomatoes (1½ cups)

Salt (1/4 tsp)

Olive oil (1 tbsp)

Canned black beans (rinsed and drained, 1 cup)

1 head of torn green leaf lettuce

1 avocado (halved, pitted and chopped)

Chopped green onions (½ cup)

Red Hot Pepper Vinaigrette

Preparation:

1. Take out the fat from pork then cut it crosswise into 1/4-inch slices.
2. Place the pork slices in a bowl. Add sage, lemon peel, cumin, salt and pepper. Toss well to coat. Leave it to stand for 10 minutes.
3. Cook the pork, half at a time over medium-high heat in a large skillet until it is slightly pink in the middle. (Cook in hot oil and turn it only once). Remove and set aside.
4. Place the lettuce on a serving plate. Top with avocado, green onions, beans and tomatoes.
5. Arrange the pork slices over salad and drizzle with some Spicy Pepper Vinaigrette.

Spicy Pepper Vinaigrette

1. Start by preheating the oven to 425 degrees F.
2. Cut 1 fresh jalapeno pepper & 1 red sweet pepper lengthwise in halves. Take out the seeds, stems and membranes. On a foil-lined baking sheet, place the pepper halves and cut sides down.
3. Bake until skin is blistered and burnt. Bring up foil around peppers to enclose. Leave it to stand until cool. Loosen edges of the skins with a sharp knife. Gently remove the skin in strips and discard.
4. Place peppers in a food processor or blender. Add 2 tbsp lime juice, 2 tbsp vinegar, 2 tbsp olive oil and 1/8 tsp of salt. Cover and process or blend until smooth.

Dinner

Beef And Plantain Kabobs With Jerk Seasoning
Ingredients:

Boneless beef sirloin steak (12 ounces)

Red wine vinegar (2 tbsp)

Cooking oil (1 tbsp)

Jamaican jerk seasoning (1 tbsp)

2 ripe plantains cut into 1-inch portions

Lime wedges (optional)

1 medium red onion (cut into wedges)

Torn salad greens (optional)

Preparation:

1. Remove fat from meat and cut it into 1-inch chunks.
2. In a small bowl, add red wine vinegar, jerk seasoning and oil. Stir together. Toss meat chunks with half of the vinegar mixture. Brush onion wedges and plantain with the remaining vinegar mixture.
3. Place skewers directly over medium coals on the rack of an uncovered grill. Grill for 15 minutes, turning occasionally. Serve with lime wedges and salad greens if desired.
4. Makes 4 servings.

Snack

½ cup of non fat fruited yogurt

1 medium apple

DAY 20
Breakfast

- 2 slice of whole wheat bread
- 1 cup of fat- free milk
- 1 tbsp of peanut butter

Lunch

Chicken & Veg Soup
Ingredients:

Reduced-sodium chicken broth (2, 14-ounce cans)

Water (2 cups)

Black pepper (1/4 tsp)

Dried whole wheat rotini, broken fusilli or twisted spaghetti (1 cup)

Vegetable pieces (e.g. chopped green or red sweet pepper, small broccoli florets, thinly sliced carrots, and/or frozen or fresh whole kernel corn, 3 cups)

Cubed cooked chicken (1 ½ cups, about 8 ounces)

Snipped fresh basil (1 tbsp)

Finely shredded Parmesan cheese (1/4 cup, 1 ounce)

Preparation:

1. Combine the broth, black pepper and water in a Dutch oven. Bring to boiling.
2. Add the pasta, stir and return to boiling. Reduce the heat, simmer and cover for 5 minutes. Add vegetables, stir.
3. Reduce heat and return to boiling. Simmer, cover until pasta and vegetables are tender. Stir in the chicken and basil. Allow to heat through.
4. Top with Parmesan cheese to serve.

5. makes 6 Servings

Dinner

Parmesan Fish & Nuts

½ of cup of Cole slaw

Parmesan Fish & Nuts
Ingredients:

1 pound of frozen or fresh orange roughly fillets

Ground pine nuts or almonds (2 tbsp)

1 beaten egg

Milk (2 tbsp)

Finely crushed rich round crackers (1/4 cup)

Grated Parmesan cheese (2 tbsp)

Dried basil, crushed (½ tsp)

Pepper (1/8 tsp)

Melted margarine or butter (2 tbsp)

Preparation:

1. Thaw fish if it is frozen. Measure fillets thickness. Cut the fish fillets into strips of 1-inch width. Rinse and use paper towels to pat dry; set aside.
2. Combine egg and milk in a shallow dish. Combine crushed crackers, pepper, Parmesan cheese, basil and groundnuts in another shallow dish.
3. Dip the fish pieces into egg mixture. Roll the fish in crumb mixture. Next, place the coated fish in a greased shallow pan.

4. Drizzle melted butter or margarine over fish. Bake, uncovered, for 10 to 15 minutes in a 500 degree F oven. (Fish flakes easily with a fork; coating also becomes golden when ready).
5. 4 Servings.

Snack

Fruit and Cheese Kabobs
Ingredients:

Honeydew melon or cantaloupe slices (4)

Monterey Jack cheese slices or reduced-fat cheddar cheese or (2 oz)

4 fresh blackberries

4whole fresh strawberries

Preparation:

1. Using 1- to 1½ -inch cookie cutters, cut shapes out of honeydew and cantaloupe slices and cheese.
2. Thread cheese and fruit onto 4 small skewers.
3. Place in a storage container and leave to chill up to 24 hours or until serving
4. Serves 2.

DAY 21
Breakfast

1 cup of fat free milk

Spicy Irish Oatmeal
Ingredients:

Water (3 cups)

Fat-free milk (3 cups)

Steel-cut oats (1 cup)

Packed brown sugar (1 tbsp)

Ground cinnamon (1/4 tsp)

Salt (1/8 tsp)

Ground allspice (1/8 tsp)

Ground nutmeg or dash ground cloves

Preparation:

1. Combine the steel-cut oats, water, allspice, brown sugar, nutmeg or cloves, cinnamon and salt in a 2-quart saucepan.
2. Bring to boiling and then reduce heat. Uncover it and let it simmer 15 minutes. Stir occasionally.
3. Serve with milk. Makes 3 cups (six ½ cup servings).

Lunch

Fireplace Beef Stew

Ingredients:

Beef chuck pot roast, boneless (1½ pounds)

Butternut squash (peeled, seeded and cut, about 2½ cups, 1 pound)

2 small onions (cut into wedges)

2 cloves minced garlic

Reduced-sodium beef broth (1, 14-ounce can)

Tomato sauce (1 8-ounce can)

Worcestershire sauce (2 tbsp)

Dry mustard (1 tsp)

Frozen Italian green beans (1 9-ounce)

Ground black pepper (1/4 tsp)

Ground allspice (1/8 tsp)

Cold water (2 tbsp)

Cornstarch (4 tsp)

Preparation:

1. Remove fat from meat and then cut it into 1-inch pieces. Next, place the meat in a quart slow cooker.
2. Add onions, garlic and squash. Stir in Worcestershire sauce, beef broth, pepper, tomato sauce, dry mustard and allspice. Cover and cook on high heat for 4 to 5 hours.
3. Combine cold water and cornstarch in a small bowl. Stir this cornstarch mixture & green beans into the mixture on the slow cooker.

4. Cover and cook until it is thickened.
5. Makes 6 servings.

Dinner

- Poached Salmon With Orange Vinaigrette
- ½ cup of wild rice
- ½ cup of steamed spinach

Poached Salmon With Orange Vinaigrette
Ingredients:

Frozen or fresh frozen salmon fillet (1½ pounds)

Finely shredded orange peel (1 tbsp)

Fresh orange juice (1/3 cup)

Balsamic vinegar or white balsamic vinegar (1/4 cup)

Finely chopped onion (2 tbsp)

Snipped fresh parsley (1 tbsp)

Snipped fresh basil (1 tbsp)

Snipped fresh mint (1 tbsp)

Salt (1/8 tsp)

Dry white wine (½ cup)

Water (½ cup)

Torn mixed greens (6 cup)

Edible flowers (optional)

Orange peel curls (optional)

Preparation:

1. Thaw frozen fish. Cut it into four pieces. Rinse and pat dry with paper towels.
2. For vinaigrette, combine orange juice, parsley, mint, onion, orange peel, basil, vinegar and salt in a screw-top container. Cover and shake thoroughly. Refrigerate until serving time.
3. In a large skillet, bring wine and water to boil. Use a wide spatula to place the fish into the boiling liquid so to prevent the pieces from overlapping. Add more water to cover fish and return to boiling.
4. Reduce heat, simmer and cover until fish flakes easily when it is tested with a fork (allow 5 to 6 minutes for each fish of ½ -inch thickness.
5. Meanwhile, divide the mixed greens into four servings. Place a salmon fillet on top greens. If desired, garnish with edible flowers and orange peel curls.
6. Serve with vinaigrette.

Snack

6 whole wheat crackers

½ cup of yogurt

DAY 22
Breakfast

1 cup of fat free milk

Buckwheat Blueberry Pancakes

Buckwheat flour (½ cup)

Whole wheat flour (½ cup)

Sugar (1 tbsp)

Baking powder (½ tsp)

Baking soda (1/4 tsp)

Salt (1/4 tsp)

Fresh or frozen blueberries, thawed (½ cup)

Frozen or refrigerated egg product (1/4 cup) or 1 egg, slightly beaten

Buttermilk or sour milk (1-1/4 cups)

Cooking oil (1 tbsp)

Vanilla (1/4 tsp)

Preparation:

1. Stir together buckwheat flour, whole wheat flour, baking powder, sugar, baking soda and salt in a medium bowl. Make a well at the center of the flour mixture and then set aside.
2. Beat egg slightly in a small bowl. Stir in oil, buttermilk and vanilla. Add all the buttermilk mixture to flour mixture. Stir just until mixed but still slightly lumpy. Add the blueberries and stir.
3. Heat a greased griddle over medium heat until some drops of water sprinkled onto griddle dance across the surface. Pour a scant 1/4 cup of batter for each pancake on the hot griddle. Spread the batter into a 4inch diameter circle.

4. Cook over medium heat until the pancakes are brown. Cook each side for 1-2 minutes.
5. Keep warm or serve immediately. Makes 6 (2-pancake) servings.

Lunch

Sea Baked Fish
Ingredients:

Olive oil (2 tsp)

1 large sliced onion

Whole tomatoes, drained & chopped (1 can, 16 oz)

1 bay leaf

1 minced clove garlic

Dry white wine (1 cup)

Reserved tomato juice, from canned tomatoes (½ cup)

Lemon juice (1/4 cup)

Orange juice (1/4 cup)

Dried thyme, crushed (½ tsp)

Fresh grated orange peel (1 tbsp)

Dried oregano, crushed (½ tsp)

Fennel seeds, crushed (1 tsp)

Dried basil, crushed (½ tsp)

Black pepper (to taste)

Fish fillets (1 lb)

Preparation:

1. In a large nonstick skillet, heat the oil. Add onion and stir- fry over moderate heat 5 until soft.
2. Add all the rest of the ingredients except fish. Stir well and simmer uncovered for 30 minutes.
3. Place fish in a 10x6-inch baking dish and cover with sauce.
4. Bake, uncovered, at 375° F until fish flakes easily.
5. 4 servings. Serving Size: 4 oz fillet with sauce

Dinner

Grilled Mixed Vegetables

Herby Peppered Sirloin Steak
Ingredients:

Catsup (2 tbsp)

Coarsely ground black pepper (½ tsp)

Snipped fresh rosemary (1 ½ tsp) or dried rosemary, crushed (½ tsp)

Snipped fresh basil (1 ½ tsp or dried basil, crushed (½ tsp)

Garlic powder (1/8 tsp)

Ground cardamom (optional, 1/8 tsp)

Boneless beef sirloin steak (1 ½ pounds)

Fresh rosemary (optional)

Grilled sweet peppers (optional)

Preparation:

1. Stir together black pepper, catsup, rosemary, garlic powder, basil and cardamom (optional). Coat the two sides of steak with the catsup mixture.
2. Grill steak uncovered for 6 minutes grill directly over medium coals. Turn the steak; grill until desired doneness. Cut into sizes.

3. Garnish with fresh rosemary and if desired, serve with grilled sweet peppers.
4. Makes 6 servings.

Snack

Rich Chips & Dip
Ingredients:

Whole wheat tortillas, red pepper and/or spinach **(2)**

Chopped fresh pineapple (2 cups)

Finely chopped red sweet pepper (½ cup)

1 sliced green onion

Lime juice (2 tbsp)

Snipped fresh cilantro (1 tbsp)

Preparation:

1. Begin by heating oven to 375 degrees F.
2. On a large baking sheet, place tortilla wedges in a single layer. Coat lightly with vegetable cooking spray.
3. Bake until crisp and golden. Set aside to cool. Store at room temperature in an airtight container for up to 3 days.
4. Stir together pineapple, green onion, cilantro, sweet red pepper and lime juice in a medium bowl. Cover and chill for about 48 hours.
5. Serve tortilla wedges with salsa. Serves 4.

DAY 23
Breakfast

Winter Fruity Crunch
Ingredients:

Assorted fresh fruit (e.g. seedless grapes, grapefruit or orange sections, cubed fresh pineapple, sliced kiwi fruit and chopped apple or pear, 4 cups)

Honey (2 tbsp)

Low-fat vanilla yogurt (2 6-ounce carton)

Low-fat granola (½ cup)

Toasted coconut (optional, 1/4 cup)

Preparation:

1. Divide fruit among 6 parfait glasses, individual dishes or tall glasses.
2. Top with yogurt and drizzle with honey.
3. Sprinkle with coconut and granola (optional)
4. serves 6

Lunch

1 side salad

Red-kidney Bean Soup
Ingredients:

Dry red kidney beans (1 pound)

Water (6 cups)

Water (8 cups)

Reduced-sodium beef broth or dry white wine (3/4 cup)

1 pound of fresh beef brisket, fat-trimmed and cut into 3/4-inch pieces

1 medium chopped green or red sweet pepper

1 medium chopped onion

4 minced cloves garlic

1 medium banana chile pepper or fresh yellow wax chile pepper

1 medium chopped tomato

1 large peeled and diced russet potato

1 ham hock

Salt (1 tsp)

Ground black pepper (½ tsp)

Preparation:

1. Combine beans and water (6cups) in a Dutch oven. Bring to boiling and reduce heat. Simmer for 1- 2 minutes. Remove from heat. Cover it and leave for 1 hour. Alternatively, place beans in water in a pan. Cover and leave to soak overnight or for 7- 8 hours in a cool place. Drain beans and rinse.
2. Return beans to oven. Add the broth or wine, 8 cups water, sweet pepper, tomato, onion, chile pepper and garlic. Bring to boiling; add ham hock and beef brisket. Return to boiling; reduce heat.
3. Cover and simmer until beans and meat are tender or for about 1 & ½ hours. Remove the ham hock and set aside to cool. Slightly mash beans. Add potato to the bean mixture. Return to boiling and reduce heat.
4. Cover and simmer for about 20 minutes until potato is tender. Once ham is cool enough, cut meat from bone and discard bone. Cut ham into pieces; stir into the bean mixture.
5. Stir in salt and black pepper.
6. 10 (1½ cup) Servings

Dinner

Poached Halibut with Peppers
Ingredients

Dry white wine or chicken broth (1½ cups)

1 cup of water

2 medium chopped yellow sweet peppers (1½ cups)

Drained capers (3 tsp)

4 minced cloves garlic

Crushed red pepper (1/4 to ½ tsp)

Basil oil or olive oil (2 tbsp)

4 halibut steaks (1½ to 13/4 lb.) or 4 cod fillets

Salt and freshly ground black pepper

Coarsely chopped fresh parsley

Preparation:
1. Combine wine, capers, water, crushed red pepper, sweet pepper and garlic for poaching liquid in a skillet and then bring to boiling. Reduce the heat, simmer, uncovered, for 6- 7 minutes, while stirring occasionally.
2. Place fish in one layer in the poaching liquid inside the skillet. Season the fish with salt and pepper. Next, spoon liquid over fish and return to simmer.
3. Cook, covered, for 4 to 6 minutes for every ½ -inch thickness of fish until the fish flakes effortlessly when tested with a fork.
4. Remove fish to platter. Pour poaching liquid to a small serving pitcher. Sprinkle cooked fish with olive oil or basil oil and some of the poaching liquid. Sprinkle it with parsley.

5. Serve with the remaining poaching liquid. serves 4

Snack

½ cup of non fat yogurt

2 Mandarins

DAY 24
Breakfast

Easy and Quick Omelet
Ingredients

Egg product (refrigerated or frozen thawed, 2 cups) or 8 eggs

Shredded reduced-fat cheddar cheese (½ cup, 2 ounces)

Snipped fresh chives, Italian parsley or chervil (2 tbsp)

Salt (1/8 tsp)

Cayenne pepper (1/8 tsp)

Torn fresh spinach or fresh baby spinach leaves (2 cups)

Red Pepper Relish (1 recipe)

Preparation:

1. Coat nonstick skillet with cooking spray. Heat the skillet over medium heat. Combine eggs, cayenne pepper, chives and salt in a large bowl. Use wire whisk or rotary beater to beat until it is frothy. Pour into skillet.
2. Use a plastic or wooden spatula to immediately stir the eggs gently but continuously until the mixture looks like small pieces of cooked egg the midst of liquid egg. Stop stirring.
3. Cook until egg is shiny and set and then sprinkle with cheese. Top with 1/4 cup of the Red Pepper Relish and 1 cup of spinach.
4. Using a spatula, lift and fold 1 side of omelet partly over filling. Arrange the rest of the spinach on a warm platter. Place omelet in platter. Top with the remaining relish.
5. Makes 4 servings.

Red Pepper Relish

1. Combine 2/3 cup of chopped red sweet pepper, 1/4 tsp black pepper, 2 tbsp of finely chopped green onion or onion and 1 tablespoon cider vinegar in a small bowl.
2. Coat a 10-inch skillet with cooking spray. Heat the skillet over medium heat.
3. Combine eggs, cayenne pepper, chives and salt in a large bowl. Beat until frothy and then pour into the skillet. Use a wooden or plastic spatula top gently and continuously stir until it looks like small cooked egg pieces surrounded by liquid egg.
4. Cook for about 60 seconds until egg is set and shiny. Sprinkle with cheese.
5. Top with 1 cup of spinach and 1/4 cup Red Pepper Relish.
6. Lift and then fold one side of omelet partly over filling. Place remaining spinach on a warm platter. Transfer the omelet to platter.
7. Top with remaining relish. Recipe makes 4 servings.

Lunch

Pappardelle Pasta & Roasted Tomatoes
Ingredients:

8 plum tomatoes, each one halved lengthwise

Olive oil (3 tbsp)

Pappardelle pasta (12 ounces)

1 minced clove garlic, minced

Salt

Freshly ground black pepper

Tomato sauce (1, 8-ounce can)

Freshly ground black pepper (1/4 tsp)

Snipped fresh thyme (1 tbsp)

Crushed red pepper (1/4 tsp)

Shaved pecorino Romano cheese (1/4 tsp)

Preparation:

1. Preheat your oven to 450 degree F. Line a baking pan with foil to roast tomatoes. Place tomatoes, cut side up, in pan. Drizzle with 1 tbsp of the oil and sprinkle with pepper and salt.
2. Roast, uncovered, in the oven for about 25 minutes or until the bottoms of tomatoes are dark brown. Take out from pan and gently halve each piece.
3. In a 4-quart Dutch oven, cook the pasta in line with package directions. Drain and set aside.
4. In the same pan, cook the garlic in the remaining 2 tbsp oil over medium heat for 35 seconds. Stir in half of the thyme, the crushed red pepper and the tomato sauce. Bring to boiling and reduce heat. Simmer, uncovered, for 1- 2 minutes.
5. Add pasta, roasted tomatoes, black pepper and remaining thyme. Heat through. Season to taste with freshly ground pepper and additional salt. Transfer to a serving dish and sprinkle with cheese.
6. Makes 4 main-dish or 8 side-dish servings.

Dinner

- 1 Whole wheat tortillas
- 1/3 cup of steamed corn
- ½ cup of steamed mixed vegetables
- Fajitas Chicken Fry

Fajitas Chicken Fry
Ingredients

Fajita seasoning mix (1 to 1.5-ounce envelope)

Water (½ cup)

Cooking oil (2 tbsp)

Skinless, boneless chicken breast halves (12 ounces, cut into 1-inch pieces)

1 medium green or yellow sweet pepper, cut into squares

1 small zucchini

Small onion (½)

2/3 cup of salsa

Chili powder (1 tsp)

Frozen whole kernel corn (½ cup)

Cooked or canned black beans, rinsed and drained (½ cup)

Nonstick spray coating

Preparation:

1. For marinade, combine water, fajita mix and oil in a medium mixing bowl. Add chicken and stir to coat. Leave to stand for 15 minutes at room temperature.
2. Spray skillet with nonstick coating. Preheat it over medium heat. Next, add sweet pepper, onion and zucchini. Cook and stir until crisp-tender. Remove from the skillet.
3. Drain the chicken and throw away marinade. Add chicken to skillet. Cook and stir until no pink remains. Bring the vegetables back to skillet. Stir together chili powder and salsa.
4. Add salsa mixture, beans and corn to skillet. Cook and stir until it is heated through.
5. Makes 4 servings.

Snack

Sparkling Stars

Ingredients:

Red, yellow, orange or blue fruit-flavored gelatin (3, 3-ounce packages)

3 envelopes unflavored gelatin

4 cups of white grape juice, apple juice or water

Preparation:

1. Stir flavored and unflavored gelatin together in a large bowl; set aside.
2. Bring the juice to boiling in a medium saucepan. Next, pour into gelatin mixture in bowl. Stir continuously until fully dissolved.
3. Pour mixture into a baking pan. Chill until gelatin is set. Cut into star shapes using a cookie cutter or cut into 1-½ -inch squares.
4. Makes 48 squares or 24 (2-inch) stars.

DAY 25
Breakfast

½ cup of fat-free yogurt

Oat With Nut Crunch Mix
Ingredients:

Brown sugar-flavored oat biscuit cereal or sweetened oat square cereal (4 cups)

Light raisins and/or dried cherries (1 cup)

Melted butter or margarine (2 tbsp)

Sliced almonds (½ cup)

Apple pie spice (½ tsp)

Dash of salt

Preparation:

1. Combine cereal and almonds in a 15x10x1-inch baking pan.
2. Stir together apple pie spice, melted butter and salt in a small bowl. Drizzle the butter mixture over the cereal mixture and toss to coat.
3. Bake for about 20 minutes in a 300 degree F oven, stirring just once during baking. Let it cool in the pan on a wire rack for 25 minutes. Stir in the dried cherries. Allow to cool completely.
4. Store in a tightly covered jar at room temperature for up to 1 week. Makes 20 servings.

Lunch

Southwest Chicken Wraps
Ingredients:

Skinless, boneless chicken breast strips (12 ounces)

Chili powder (½ tsp)

Garlic powder (1/4 tsp)

Nonstick cooking spray

1 small red, green or yellow sweet pepper (seeded and cut into strips)

Bottled reduced-calorie ranch salad dressing (2 tbsp)

Whole wheat, plain flour warmed tortillas, tomato or jalapeno (2, 10-inch)

Fresh Tasty Salsa (½ cup)

Reduced-fat shredded cheddar cheese (1/3 cup)

Preparation:

1. Sprinkle chili powder and garlic powder on chicken strips. Coat a nonstick skillet with nonstick spray and heat over medium-high heat.
2. Cook the chicken and sweet pepper strips in over medium heat until pepper strips are tender and chicken is no longer pink. Drain and toss with salad dressing.
3. Divide pepper mixture and chicken between warmed tortillas. Top with Fresh Tasty Salsa and cheese. Roll them up and cut in half.
4. Wrap tortillas tightly in foil to warm it. Heat in a 350 degrees F oven until heated through.
5. Fresh Tasty Salsa: combine 2 seeded and chopped tomatoes, 1/4 cup of chopped green or yellow sweet pepper, 2- 3 tsp snipped fresh cilantro, /4 cup of finely chopped red onion, 1/8 teaspoon salt, 1 ½ 2 teaspoon minced garlic, few drops of bottled hot pepper sauce (optional) and a dash of black pepper. Cover and chill for 3

days or serve immediately. Stir before serving. Recipe makes 1 2/3 cups.

Dinner

Crusted- Parmesan Fish

½ cup of cooked cauliflower

½ cup of cooked okra

Crusted- Parmesan Fish Recipe
Ingredients

Skinless cod fillets (4, 1½ lb)

Panko bread crumbs (1/3 cup)

Finely shredded Parmesan cheese (1/4 cup)

Carrots thinly cut (3 cups)

Butter (1 tbsp)

Ground ginger (3/4 tsp)

Mixed fresh salad greens

Preparation:

1. Begin by preheating oven to 450 degrees F. Coat a baking sheet lightly with nonstick cooking spray. Rinse fish and pat dry. Place on baking sheet. Season with pepper and salt.
2. Stir together crumbs and cheese in small bowl; sprinkle on fish. For each ½ -inch thickness of fish, bake, without covering for 4 to 6 minutes until fish flakes easily when tested with a fork and crumbs are golden.
3. Bring ½ cup of water to boiling in a large skillet; add carrots. Reduce the heat. Cover and cook for 5 minutes. Uncover and cook for 2 minutes longer. Add butter and ginger and then toss.
4. Serve with greens. Serves 4.

Snack

1 slice of whole wheat bread

1 tsp of almond butter

DAY 26
Breakfast

- 1 slice of whole wheat bread
- ½ cup of plain yogurt
- ½ cup of blueberries
- ½ cup of home-squeezed orange without sugar

Lunch

- Chicken Breasts With Summer Squash
- 1 Small Mixed Garden Salad

Chicken Breasts With Summer Squash Recipe
Ingredients:

Skinless, boneless chicken breast halves (4 medium-sized, about 3/4 pound total)

Olive oil (1 tbsp)

Pesto (2 tbsp)

Yellow summer squash and/or finely chopped zucchini (2 cups)

Shredded Asiago or Parmesan cheese (2 tbsp)

Preparation:

1. Over medium heat, cook chicken in hot oil for 4 minutes in a large skillet.
2. Turn chicken and add squash and/or zucchini. Cook for another 4 to 6 minutes (170 degrees F) until the chicken is soft and no longer pink and squash is crisp-tender. Gently stir squash once or twice.
3. Transfer squash and chicken to 4 dinner plates. Spread the pesto over chicken and then sprinkle with Asiago or Parmesan cheese.
4. Makes 4 servings.

Dinner

Seafood Kebab

½ cup of couscous

Seafood Kebab
Ingredients:

1 pound skinless fresh fish fillets

Frozen or fresh medium shrimp in shells (½ pound)

Olive oil (1/4 cup)

4 minced cloves garlic

2 medium fennel bulbs

Lemon juice (3 tbsp)

Snipped fresh oregano (3 tbsp)

Salt (1/4 tsp)

Preparation:

1. Rinse the fish fillets and use paper towels to pat dry. Cut them into 1-inch cubes. Set aside. Thaw the shrimp, if frozen. Peel & devein the shrimp but leave the tails intact. Rinse &pat dry shrimp; Set aside.

2. Cut off and throw away upper stalks of fennel bulbs but reserve some of the leafy fronds. Snip 2 tbsp of fronds to be used for the marinade. Take out any wilted outer layers from the bulbs. Next, cut off a slim slice from the base of each bulb. Wash and cut each of the bulbs lengthwise into six wedges. Cover and cook wedges in some boiling water for about 5 minutes, then drain.

3. Place fennel wedges, fish cubes and shrimp in a plastic bag set in a bowl. For marinade, stir together olive oil, snipped fennel fronds, oregano, lemon juice, garlic and salt. Pour over seafood and fennel wedges. Close the self-

sealing bag. Marinate in the refrigerator for up to 2 hours, turning now and then.

4. Drain fennel wedges, fish cubes and shrimp discarding marinade. Thread shrimp, fish cubes and fennel wedges on skewers.

5. Place directly over medium-hot coals on a greased rack of a grill. Grill, uncovered (turning often) until fish flakes when it is tested with a fork and the shrimp turn opaque. This recipe makes 6 servings.

Snack

Maple Sugary Corn

1 medium banana

Maple Sugary Corn Recipe
Ingredients:

Canola oil (2 tbsp)

Non-popped popcorn kernels (½ cup)

Maple sugar (1/4 cup)

Kosher salt (½ tsp)

Preparation:

1. Heat oil in a pan over medium-high heat. Add sugar, popcorn and salt to saucepan; cover and cook until kernels begin to pop. Continue cooking for 2 minutes, constantly shaking pan to prevent burning.
2. When popping reduces, remove pan from heat. Leave it to stand, covered until popping stops.

DAY 27
Breakfast

- Whole wheat pancake (no syrup)
- 1/4 cup of fat- free cottage cheese
- 1 cup of fresh pineapple

Lunch

- spiced-laced chicken
- ½ cup of steamed green beans
- 1 cup of raw spinach with fat free salad dressing

Spiced-Laced Chicken Recipe
Ingredients:

16 skinless, boneless chicken breast halves (5 lbs)

Packed brown sugar (½ cup)

Paprika (2 tbsp)

Salt (2 tsp)

Ground coriander (2 tsp)

Ground black pepper (1 tsp)

Garlic powder (1 tsp)

Cayenne pepper (½ tsp)

Cooking oil (2 tbsp)

Preparation:

1. Combine brown sugar, salt, paprika, coriander, black pepper, cayenne pepper and garlic powder in small bowl. Brush the chicken with oil.

2. Sprinkle spice on both sides of the chicken. Use the fingers to gently rub in the spice mixture. Place on 15x10x1-inch baking pans. Next, refrigerate the chicken for 15 minutes and then preheat oven to 400 degrees F.
3. Bake chicken breasts, uncovered, one at a time at 170 degrees F until it is no longer pink. (Cover and refrigerate the second pan of chicken while baking the first pan.)
4. Leave chicken to cool. Wrap chicken breasts individually in waxed paper.
5. Divide the wrapped chicken among two freezer bags. Remove air from bags. Label them and freeze for up to 4 months.
6. Thaw and use for other recipes.

Dinner

- Marinated Pork Fillet Steak
- ½ cup of cooked asparagus
- ½ cup of cooked butternut squash

Marinated Pork Fillet Steak Recipe

Ingredients:

1-pound pork tenderloins (6)

Nipped fresh parsley (½ cup)

1 750-milliliter bottle dry white wine

Olive oil (½ cup)

Nipped fresh basil (1/4 cups)

White wine Worcestershire sauce (1/4 cup)

Cloves garlic, minced (6, 1 tbsp)

Salt (1 tsp)

Cracked black pepper (1 tsp)

Champagne or honey mustard

Preparation:

1. Place pork in rectangular baking dishes. Stir together the wine, Worcestershire sauce, oil, parsley, basil, salt, garlic and pepper in a large bowl. Pour over the pork evenly. Cover for about 24 hours to chill.
2. Preheat the oven to 450 degree F. Drain pork and discard marinade. Arrange pork in a large roasting pan. Roast for 30 to 35 minutes uncovered. Cover and let it stand for 10 minutes.
3. Transfer to a cutting board and slice tenderloin thinly. Arrange in a storage container. Cover and leave to chill for 4- 24 hours.
4. Arrange on serving platters to serve. Serve with honey mustard or champagne

Snack

Watermelon Wedges With Honey & Lime
Ingredients:

Freshly squeezed lime juice (½ cup)

Clover honey (3 tbsp)

Chilled watermelon, quartered (3 slices, 1-inch-thick)

Preparation:

1. Whisk the honey and lime juice together in a bowl until the honey dissolves.
2. On a large platter, arrange the watermelon wedges and drizzle equally with the lime-honey dressing.
3. Serve immediately.

DAY 28
Breakfast

1 cup of fat-free milk

Pecan Oatmeal with Dried Cherry
Ingredients:

Water (3 cups)

Fat-free milk (3 cups)

Whole oats (not instant, 2 cups)

Coarsely chopped dried cherries (½ cup)

Salt (½ tsp)

Brown sugar (5 tbsp)

Butter (1 tbsp)

Ground cinnamon (1/4 tsp)

Vanilla extract (1/4 tsp)

Toasted chopped pecans (2 tbsp)

Preparation:

1. Bring to boil, the water, fat-free milk, oats, cherries and salt. Reduce the heat and simmer. Stir occasionally until thickened.
2. Take out from heat. Stir in 4 tbsp of brown sugar and butter, cinnamon and vanilla extract.
3. In each of 6 bowls, spoon 1 cup of oatmeal. Sprinkle well with pecans and the remaining tablespoon of brown sugar.
4. It's ready to eat.

Lunch

½ cup of cooked cabbage

½ cup of steamed asparagus

Baked Chilies Chicken Recipe
Ingredients:

Cornmeal (3 tbsp)

6 skinless, boneless chicken breast halves

All-purpose flour (1/3 cup)

Ground red pepper (1/4 tsp)

1 egg

Water (1 tbsp)

Whole green chile peppers cut in half (1, 4-ounce can. 6 pieces total)

Monterey Jack cheese (2 ounces) cut into six 2x½ -inch sticks

Snipped fresh cilantro or fresh parsley (2 tbsp)

Black pepper (1/4 tsp)

Melted butter or margarine (2 tbsp)

Green or red salsa (1, 8-ounce jar)

Preparation:

1. Place half chicken breast between 2 pieces of plastic wrap. With the flat side of a meat mallet, lightly pound the meat into a rectangle of about 1/8 inch thick. Remove the plastic wrap.
2. Combine the ground red pepper, cornmeal and flour in a shallow dish.
3. In another shallow dish, place egg and lightly beat to combine.

4. Place a chile pepper half on a piece of chicken near an edge. (Do it for each roll). Place a stick of cheese on the chile pepper near an edge.
5. Drizzle some of the parsley or cilantro and black pepper. Fold the sides in, roll up, beginning from edge with cheese. Use wooden toothpicks to secure.
6. Dip the rolls in egg mixture and coat with cornmeal mixture. In a shallow baking pan, place rolls, seam sides down. Drizzle with butter.
7. Bake without covering in a 375 degree oven until chicken is no longer pink (170 degrees F). Take out toothpicks.
8. Meanwhile, heat the salsa and serve over chicken. Garnish with additional cilantro if desired. Makes: 6 servings

Dinner

Hot Tilapia With Lemon & Asparagus
Ingredients:

Asparagus, tough ends trimmed & cut into 1-inch pieces (2 pounds)

Chili powder (2 tbsp)

Garlic, powder (½ tsp)

Salt, divided (½ tsp)

Tilapia or other white fish fillets (1pound)

Extra-virgin olive oil (2 tbsp)

Lemon juice (3 tbsp)

Preparation:

1. In a large saucepan, bring 1 inch of water to boil. Put the asparagus in a steamer basket and place in the pan. Cover it and steam for about 4 minutes until it is tender-crisp. Spread out on a plate to cool.

2. Combine garlic powder, 1/4 teaspoon of salt and chili powder on a plate.
3. To coat, sprinkle fillets in the spice mixture.
4. In a large nonstick skillet, heat oil over medium-high heat. Add the fish and cook for 5 to 7 minutes until opaque in the center.
5. Divide among 4 plates and immediately add the remaining1/4 tsp asparagus and salt, the lemon juice to the pan and then cook. Stir constantly for about 2 minutes until the asparagus is coated and also heated through. Serve asparagus with the fish. Serves 4.

Snack

Fiesta Rolls
Ingredients:

Fresh poblano peppers (2 large)

Red sweet peppers (2 medium)

½ of an 8-ounce tub

Plain fat-free cream cheese (½ cup)

Fresh cilantro (1 tbsp)

Lime juice (2 tsp)

Ground red pepper (1/8 tsp)

2 minced cloves garlic

7-or 8-inch flour tortillas (4)

Preparation:

1. To roast sweet peppers and poblano, halve peppers and take out stems, seeds and membranes.
2. On a foil-lined baking sheet, place the peppers, cut sides down
3. Bake in a 425 degrees F oven until the skin is bubbly and browned.
4. Wrap up the peppers in the foil and let it stand until cool.

5. Use a paring knife to gently and slowly pull off the skin. Cut peppers into thin strips.
6. Stir together the cilantro, cream cheese, ground red pepper, lime juice and garlic. Spread tortillas with the cream cheese mixture.
7. Lay sweet pepper and poblano strips over the cream cheese mixture. Roll tortillas up.
8. Wrap with plastic wrap and refrigerate for about 6 hours.
9. Unwrap and slice diagonally into 1 1/4-inch slices.
10. Makes 8 to 10 servings (about 24 pieces).

Made in the USA
San Bernardino, CA
18 April 2018